TACKLING DIAPER RASH

Home Solutions for Babies' Comfort: Diaper Rash Signs and Natural Remedies

CARL JUAN

Table of Contents

Introductory

Babies and young children frequently have diaper rash because of their sensitive skin. Diaper dermatitis is another name for this condition. Redness, irritation, and inflammation of the skin in the diaper area (the buttocks, genitalia, and inner thighs) are the hallmarks of a diaper rash. A baby's delicate skin is easily irritated and damaged by prolonged contact with moisture, pee, and feces, which can lead to diaper rash.

Diaper rash has a number of common causes and contributors.

• Diapers that have been wet or soiled for a long time can cause skin to become delicate and prone to irritation.

• Diaper rash can be made worse by friction caused by the diaper rubbing against the baby's skin.

• Redness and irritation from chafing can be brought on by the tightness or friction of diapers or elastic leg openings.

• Diaper rash can be made worse by yeast or fungal infections, which thrive in the warm, moist environment of a diaper.

The following are some measures parents and caregivers can take to cure and prevent diaper rash:

• Make sure the skin is dry and clean before putting on a fresh diaper, and change diapers often.

• Apply a protective barrier lotion or ointment, such as zinc oxide, to your skin to produce a layer that will keep moisture out.

• Make sure the diaper fits snugly, but not too tightly, to reduce the risk of irritation.

• Allow air exposure: Take your infant out of diapers for short periods of time to let his or her skin breathe and recover.

• Use fragrance-free wipes and mild, hypoallergenic products to clean the diaper region to prevent irritation.

Consult a doctor or healthcare provider for additional examination and treatment of diaper rash if it is severe, persistent, or accompanied by indications of infection. To treat yeast or bacterial infections, they could suggest medicinal lotions or ointments. Care and cleanliness go a long way toward alleviating diaper rash.

CHAPTER ONE
Diaper Rash's Root Causes

There is no single cause for diaper rash, and in most cases, several variables work together. The most typical reasons for a diaper rash are:

1. Diaper rash is often caused by a baby's skin coming into prolonged contact with wet or soiled diapers. The baby's skin may become more delicate and prone to discomfort if it comes into contact with urine or feces.

2. Friction and chafing: The diaper itself, especially if it is overly tight or scrapes against the baby's skin, can generate friction and chafing, which can lead to skin irritation.

3. Infections caused by yeasts or fungi like Candida thrive in the warm, wet conditions found inside a diaper. Rashes made worse by these illnesses can be quite irritating.

4. Sensitivity to particular diaper materials or chemicals: Some newborns may have a sensitivity or allergy to the materials, scents, or chemicals in disposable diapers, wipes, or the detergents used to wash cloth diapers. This might cause irritation to the skin.

5. The introduction of solid foods, in particular, can cause a shift in the makeup of a baby's bowel movements, which may irritate the skin.

6. Antibiotics: Antibiotics may increase a baby's susceptibility to yeast infections by upsetting the delicate balance of natural microorganisms that live on their skin.

7. Diaper rash can be exacerbated by an infant's increased production of acidic urine and feces, which can occur during teething or illness.

8. Diarrhea: Frequent or severe diarrhea might increase the chance of diaper rash because of the increased contact with feces.

9. The introduction of new meals can alter the makeup of a baby's stool, which may increase the likelihood that it will cause skin irritation.

10. The risk of diaper rash is greatly increased if diapers are not changed as often as recommended.

It's important to remember that there's a wide range in the severity of diaper rashes. Some may start out mild and respond well to preventative measures, while others may worsen to the point where they are painful and require medical attention. Seek medical attention for diagnosis and treatment if a diaper rash continues, worsens, or is accompanied by evidence of infection like pus, blisters, or open sores.

Diaper Rash Treatment Is Crucial.

Diaper rash can have both short-term and long-term impacts on a baby's comfort, health, and well-being, making it essential that it be treated.

- Diaper rash can cause pain and discomfort for your infant. It's common for the diaper area to get red, irritated, and sore due to this, making it uncomfortable for the infant to sleep, play, or feel at ease. The baby's quality of life can be enhanced by acting quickly to alleviate this pain.

- **Prevention of Infection:** Diaper rash can make the baby's skin more susceptible to secondary infections, such as yeast or bacterial infections. Treating the rash as soon as possible can stop an infection from spreading and becoming life-threatening.

• Reduce the Risk of Permanent Skin Changes and Scarring Severe or persistent diaper rash can cause permanent skin changes in both appearance and feel if left untreated. If treated in a timely manner, the potential for such enduring consequences can be mitigated.

• The sooner a diaper rash is addressed, the quicker it usually heals. Avoiding the rash's treatment or putting it off can lengthen the time it takes to feel well.

5. Diaper rash is an irritant that, if left untreated, can intensify, resulting in more pain and a longer

healing time. The severity of the rash might be reduced with the right treatment.

• A baby's health and happiness are directly related to their quality of life. Maintaining their standard of living and avoiding unnecessary pain can be accomplished by quick treatment of diaper rash.

• The stress that diaper rash can cause for parents and caregivers is reduced. Addressing the issue early and properly helps lessen stress and worry connected to caring for an uncomfortable or irritable baby.

•Improved Parent-Child Bond: A baby that is comfortable and happy is more likely to have a positive interaction with their caretakers. Diaper rash treatment is a great way for parents to bond with their children.

• Good hygiene practices, such as changing diapers frequently and giving the diaper area a thorough washing, can be established if parents and caregivers act quickly when they notice signs of a diaper rash. These routines can help keep diaper rash at bay.

- In extreme circumstances, subsequent infections caused by untreated diaper rash might cause serious health problems. You're doing your part to ensure your baby's health by preventing and treating diaper rash.

In conclusion, treating diaper rash quickly is important not just because it helps the infant feel better, but also because it prevents further issues, creates a more pleasant environment for the baby, and eases the burden on the caregiver. It's crucial to a baby's health and well-being, so make sure you're doing it!

CHAPTER TWO
How to Spot the Warning Signs

Understanding the causes and symptoms of diaper rash will allow you to provide your infant with the care they need faster. Diaper rash typically manifests with these symptoms:

• Redness is the most obvious and typical symptom of a diaper rash. The skin could look red, pink, or irritated.

• Symptoms of irritation include redness, heat, and swelling at the site of the problem.

•   Raised Bumps or Pimples: Sometimes, you may detect raised red bumps or little pimples in the diaper area.

• **Swelling:** The skin in the diaper area may appear swollen or puffy.

•   Babies can show signs of discomfort or tenderness around the diaper area. They may be difficult to change diapers or soothe when they are cranky.

• Diaper area skin may be warmer to the touch than other areas of the body.

• In rare situations, you may discover that your child's skin in the diaper area is peeling or flaking.

• Diaper rash is caused by the diaper rubbing against the skin and irritating it more.

• Diaper rash's worst case scenario is the development of open sores or ulcers that may ooze fluid or pus.

• Small, raised, red or white lumps at the rash's margins are a telltale sign of a yeast or fungal infection, and the rash may spread beyond the diaper area onto the baby's legs and tummy.

• Broken skin or bleeding are both extremely unusual side effects of severe diaper rash.

• Putrid Scent: Urine and feces breaking down on inflamed skin can cause a strong, unpleasant stench, which is a common symptom of diaper rash.

It's crucial to pay special attention to your baby's diaper area throughout each diaper change to notice any signs of diaper rash early. Keep in aware that diaper rash can range from moderate to severe, and the severity can alter fast. As soon as you see any redness or irritation, you should take action to stop it from getting worse.

Additionally, it's vital to discern between a basic diaper rash and other illnesses, such as a yeast infection or bacterial infection. Seek medical attention for an accurate diagnosis and treatment if you feel the rash is not improving with home care, is spreading, or appears infected (with indications like pus, blisters, or open sores).

Reasons Why Babies Get Diaper Rash

Diaper rashes are common in infants because of the delicate nature of their skin and the factors involved in changing their diapers. Common explanations include:

1. Wet or soiled diapers left on for too long are the most common cause of diaper rash. The baby's skin can become more delicate and prone to discomfort if it comes into contact with urine or feces.

2. Skin irritation and chafing can be caused by the diaper itself if it is overly tight or if it scrapes against the baby's skin. This might cause irritation to the skin.

3. Infections caused by yeasts or fungi, like Candida, thrive in the warm, wet conditions found inside a diaper. Rashes made worse by these illnesses can be quite irritating.

4. Material Sensitivity some infants may be hypersensitive or allergic to the dyes, perfumes, or chemicals used in disposable diapers. Even if properly laundered, cloth diapers have a risk of irritating sensitive skin.

5. Diaper rash can be caused by using soaps and wipes that are too abrasive or have strong fragrances when changing a baby's diaper.

6. Diaper rash can be exacerbated by the use of antibiotics, which can alter the composition of beneficial skin microbes and leave a newborn more susceptible to yeast infections.

7. Diet: Changes in a baby's diet, such as introducing solid foods or a new food that the infant may be sensitive to, might affect the composition of their bowel movements, perhaps making them more irritating to the skin.

8. Diaper rash can be made worse by a baby's increased production of acid in their urine and feces if they are teething or sick.

9. Diarrhea: Frequent or severe diarrhea might increase the chance of diaper rash because of the increased contact with feces.

10. The risk of diaper rash is greatly increased if diapers are not changed as often as recommended.

Keep in mind that there is a wide range in the severity of diaper rashes. Some may start out mild and respond well to preventative measures, while others may worsen to the point where they are painful and require medical attention. It is crucial to see a doctor if a diaper rash lasts more than a few days,

gets worse, or is accompanied by
other symptoms of illness.

CHAPTER THREE
Diapering Strategies and Preventative Measures

Maintaining your baby's comfort and skin health depends on your diligence in preventing diaper rash and using correct diapering procedures. For better protection and diapering results, consider these suggestions:

Prevention:

1. Regular Diaper Changes: It is recommended that you change your baby's diaper every two to three hours, or as soon as it becomes moist or dirty. One of the best preventative methods is to make sure the diaper region stays dry.

2. At each diaper change, gently cleanse your baby's diaper region with a mild, fragrance-free baby wipe or with warm water and a soft cloth. Wipes containing alcohol, perfumes, or any other allergens should be avoided.

3. After washing, make sure the skin around the diaper region is totally dry by patting it with a clean, dry cloth before applying a new diaper.

4. Use a barrier lotion (often a zinc oxide-based cream) to prevent diaper rash from occurring on your baby's skin. This can reduce the likelihood that your skin will be harmed by water vapor.

5. Diaper Choice: Go for something that fits well and is made to keep the baby dry. Cloth diapers or disposables that are hypoallergenic and fragrance-free may be the best option for your baby's comfort.

6. Give your infant some time out of diapers every day to let their skin breathe. Put a waterproof cushion or towel down for them to sit on.

7. Overly tight diapers can irritate the skin by rubbing against it, so it's important to get the fit just right. Examine the waist and the length of the legs to make sure they fit properly.

8.Follow the manufacturer's recommendations for washing and using cloth diapers. To avoid diaper rash, be careful to clean and sanitize the diapers thoroughly.

Methods for Efficient Changing of Diapers:

1. Have everything you need close at hand before beginning the diaper change. This includes a fresh diaper, wipes, a clean cloth or tissue, and a diaper rash cream or ointment.

2. First and foremost, always keep one hand on your baby to protect them from rolling or falling while changing them. This includes when they are on a changing table or other safe surface.

3. Use soft, upward strokes when wiping to prevent transferring feces or urine to the vaginal area. Girls, please wipe from front to back to avoid spreading germs.

4. Proper Disposal Entails rolling the dirty diaper and securing it with the tabs. Do not leave soiled diapers laying around, as this might cause unpleasant scents and make your infant uncomfortable.

5. Allow the diaper area to air dry or pat it gently with a clean towel before applying a new diaper.

6. Make sure the skin is completely dry before applying a thin layer of diaper rash cream or ointment to act as a barrier and prevent further irritation.

7. Secure Diaper Snugly: Fasten the diaper securely but not too firmly, ensuring there is ample area for breathability.

8. Make sure there are no gaps around the legs and waist, and that the diaper fits snugly but not too tightly.

Diaper rash can be avoided and your baby's skin can be kept healthy and comfortable if you use these preventative steps and good diapering procedures. Diaper rashes can be easily treated if caught early and given the proper care and attention.

CHAPTER FOUR
Remedy for Diaper Rash

Babies frequently experience the discomfort of a diaper rash, but this common problem can be properly treated. Diaper rash can be treated in the following ways:

1. Don't let the dust and moisture settle:

Every two to three hours is a good rule of thumb for changing a baby's diaper, but you should do it as soon as it gets wet or soiled.

• Wipe the diaper area down with warm water and a soft cloth or mild, fragrance-free baby wipes.

Wipes containing alcohol or perfumes should be avoided.

2. Clear the Air:

• Allow your infant to have some diaper-free time to let the skin air out and dry.

3. Diaper rash can be treated with a cream or ointment.

• Use a thick coating of ointment or cream designed to prevent diaper rash, preferably one that contains zinc oxide. These items aid in preventing moisture from penetrating the epidermal barrier.

If you want to keep the rash from getting infected, you should apply the medication with a clean, dry hand or a disposable applicator.

4. Loosen Up Those Diapers!

• Overly tight diapers can irritate the skin by rubbing against it, so it's important to get the fit just right.

• Check the diaper's waist and leg holes to make sure they are a good fit.

5. Make the Most of Cloth Diapers:

• Cloth diapers should be washed and rinsed well to remove any detergent residue before use. If you need to, use a diaper liner.

6. If necessary, adjust your infant's diet by:

• If you suspect that your child's diaper rash is due to their food, talk to their pediatrician about making any necessary adjustments.

7. Ointments and Creams Available at the Drugstore:

• Hydrocortisone-containing and other over-the-counter lotions and ointments may provide temporary relief from inflammation and irritation. Before giving these to your kid, though, you should talk to the pediatrician.

8. You Should See a Pediatrician

• Consult a pediatrician if the diaper rash is severe, persistent, or accompanied by infection symptoms (such as open sores, pus, blisters, or fever). Antifungal or antibiotic ointments may be prescribed for your infant.

9. Eliminate the Potential for a Food Allergy or Intolerance

• Diaper rash can be exacerbated by food allergies or sensitivities in some babies. Talk to your child's doctor if you have concerns that this might be the case.

10. Take Care of Your Hygiene:

• Every time you change your baby's diaper, be sure to provide special attention to the genital area.

• Avoid using fragrant items or harsh washes in the diaper region, since they might irritate the skin.

11. Wait It Out:

• It could be a while before a diaper rash clears up. Treatment and preventative measures should be maintained until the rash has completely cleared up.

To properly manage diaper rash, remember that prevention is crucial. You can lessen the chances of recurring diaper rashes by using safe diapering practices and practicing basic hygiene. If the rash does not improve with home treatment or if you have any other concerns, you should see a pediatrician for advice and to rule out more serious causes.

Natural and Home-Based Solutions

Diaper rash can be treated in a number of ways, including with home remedies and natural treatments. Keep in mind that while these techniques can be helpful for moderate cases of diaper rash, it is crucial to see a doctor if the rash is severe, persistent, or shows signs of infection. Diaper rash can be treated with these all-natural methods:

1. Take an Oatmeal Soak:

• Soothing inflamed skin with colloidal oatmeal. Let your baby soak in a bath containing oatmeal for 10 to 15 minutes. Keep in mind that hot water might aggravate skin irritation, so use caution.

2. Olive Oil:

• Smear some coconut oil on the injured spot. Coconut oil is a great moisturizer and natural antibacterial and antifungal.

3. The Healing Power of Aloe Vera Gel

• Without any added chemicals or scents, pure aloe vera gel can help calm and mend aggravated skin. Rub a little bit into the irritated skin.

4. A few drops of breast milk can be applied to the sore spot if you're breastfeeding. Breast milk includes antibodies and natural healing qualities.

5. Drinking Chamomile Tea:

• Make some chamomile tea and set it aside to cool. After the tea has cooled, apply it to the rash with a cotton ball or cloth. The calming and anti-inflammatory effects of chamomile are well-known.

6. Sodium bicarbonate, or baking soda:

• Add a teaspoon of baking soda to a small dish of warm water to produce a paste. Use this paste to treat the rash, and then wash it off with warm water once it has set for a few minutes. Baking soda can reduce inflammation by neutralizing acidic pH levels.

7. Live-Culture Yogurt:

• Some parents have reported success in treating their child's rash with a topical application of plain, unsweetened probiotic yogurt containing live cultures. Before giving your baby this treatment, check for milk allergies.

8. What It Is:

• To reduce swelling and inflammation, try using witch hazel, a natural astringent. Use a cotton swab to apply a small amount and dab it gently into the rash.

9. Cornstarch:

• After washing and drying the diaper region completely, a light dusting of cornstarch can help prevent leaks. However, excessive use may promote fungal growth, so moderation is key.

10. Gentle Heat:

• For a few minutes, multiple times a day, apply a warm, wet washcloth to the rash. As a result, the area will feel cleaner and calmer.

Make sure your kid doesn't have an allergic response by first testing any new medication on a small area of skin. In the event that the diaper rash gets worse, doesn't get better, or exhibits signs of infection, medical attention should be sought. It's also important to keep up with excellent hygiene habits and stick to a routine for changing diapers to avoid any more irritation.

CHAPTER FIVE
Protecting Your Infant's Skin

Taking good care of your baby's skin is crucial to their happiness, health, and development. For healthy newborn skin, remember these guidelines:

1. Soft Scrubbing:

• When bathing your infant, use lukewarm water and gentle, fragrance-free baby soap. If you have sensitive skin, I wouldn't recommend using perfumed or harsh soaps.

• Newborns should only be bathed twice or three times a week because frequent bathing might dry up their skin.

2. Do Not Rub:

• Use a gentle towel to gently dry your baby's skin after a bath. You should not rub your skin, as this can cause irritation.

3. Moisturize:

• Moisturize your baby's skin with a mild, hypoallergenic, fragrance-free lotion, especially after a bath. This aids in retaining moisture and warding off dryness.

4. Care for the Diaper Area:

• Make sure the diaper region is clean and dry by changing diapers often.

At each diaper change, clean the diaper region with a gentle, fragrance-free baby wipe or with warm water and a soft cloth.

Diaper rash can be prevented and treated by using a barrier cream or ointment on the skin around the diaper.

5. Shade from the Sun:

• Babies younger than six months should not be exposed to direct sunlight. Cover the infant with light clothing and a sun umbrella when you go outside.

Babies older than six months should have their exposed skin protected with a broad-spectrum sunscreen with an SPF of at least 30.

6. Wear Protective Attire

• Dress your infant in comfortable, breathable fabrics like cotton. Stay away from anything that can scrape or irritate your skin.

• Keep your kid from getting too hot or too cold by dressing him or her appropriately for the weather.

regular checks. Deal with problems as soon as possible.

12. Cut down on bath time and use milder soaps:

• Do not soak in the tub for too long, as this can wash away the skin's natural oils. Use gentle, fragrance-free baby soaps.

13. Advice from a Doctor:

• Seek medical attention or a pediatrician if your child develops a skin condition, rash, or illness that worries you.

Keep in mind that your baby's skin may have specific demands because no two babies have identical skin. If you follow these instructions, your baby's skin will stay healthy and you'll both have a better time.

Aside from Baby Bottoms

Diaper rash isn't the only skin issue you'll need to worry about when caring for your infant. Keeping your baby's skin healthy involves these additional measures:

1. In the Tub:

• Take baths with lukewarm water and fragrance-free baby soap. Bathe your infant 2-3 times a week throughout the first few months, gradually increasing the frequency as they develop. Excessive bathing can deplete the skin of its natural oils.

• To avoid skin dryness, limit your bathing time to no more than 10 minutes.

After drying your infant off from a bath, pat him or her dry with a soft towel.

2. Moisturize:

• Apply a light, hypoallergenic, fragrance-free moisturizer to your baby's skin, especially after bathing. This helps lock in moisture and avoid dryness.

3. Keep an eye out for skin issues beyond diaper rash, like eczema or cradle cap. For advice on how to handle these situations, speak with a pediatrician.

4. Shade from the Sun:

• Lightweight long-sleeved clothing, a wide-brimmed hat, and sunglasses are all great ways to shield your infant from the sun's damaging UV rays.

Apply a broad-spectrum sunscreen with an SPF of at least 30 to the skin of infants older than six months. Reapply sunscreen every two hours and put it on 15-30 minutes before heading outside.

5. Attire Appropriately:

• Keep your kid from getting too hot or too cold by dressing him or her appropriately for the weather. Wear multiple layers in chilly weather and airy, lightweight garments when it's warm out.

6. Cut Your Nails:

• Trim your baby's nails regularly to avoid any scratches.

7. Allergens and Fragrances:

• Avoid using strongly scented goods around your infant, including perfumes and air fresheners.

To reduce your contact with allergies, choose laundry detergent and fabric softener that are hypoallergenic and fragrance-free.

8. Adjusting the Ambient Temperature:

• Don't let the baby's room get too hot or too cold; instead, keep it at a steady, comfortable temperature. Keep the room at a comfortable temperature with the aid of a baby monitor.

9. Regular Skin Exams:

• Be on the lookout for any rashes, irritations, or strange marks on your baby's skin by performing regular checks. If you have any skin problems, it's important to consult a doctor right once.

10. Eating Well:

• If your baby has begun on solids, ensuring they have a balanced diet with a range of fruits, vegetables, and whole grains to improve general health, including skin health.

11. Hydration:

In hot weather, it's especially important to keep your infant hydrated to avoid dehydration and skin irritation.

12. See Your Child's Pediatrician:

• Seek expert advice from a doctor or healthcare practitioner if you or your child experiences any skin problems, persistent rashes, or signs of infection.

Maintaining a regular skincare routine, keeping an eye out for any skin issues, and making sure your infant is comfortable and protected from external influences all contribute to healthy skin care for your baby. Because every baby has different skin, it's important to personalize your baby's skincare routine.

Conclusion

Maintaining your baby's health, comfort, and well-being includes taking care of their skin. Diaper rash is just the beginning of what needs to be done to ensure proper skincare, which includes things like regular skin checks, mild washing, moisturizing, sun protection, dressing for the weather, and more. If you pay close attention to your baby's specific needs and adhere to these suggestions, your baby's skin should remain healthy and irritant-free.

To avoid developing skin sensitivities or allergies, it's best to stick to gentle, hypoallergenic products, steer clear of anything with a strong chemical scent, and proceed with caution when selecting a laundry detergent. In addition, if you have questions about how to treat a specific skin issue or worry, it's best to talk to a doctor.

Establishing and maintaining a good skincare routine for your infant and paying close attention to any changes in their skin health will go a long way toward ensuring their comfort and happiness, which in turn will promote healthy development.

THE END